Carbs & Cals APP

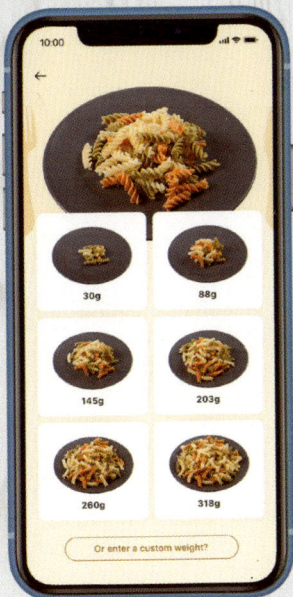

Try...

★ F... (with option to upgrade)

★ The **visual way** to count your carbs and calories, at home or on-the-go!

★ Over 130,000 foods inc **NEW barcode scanner**, brands & restaurants

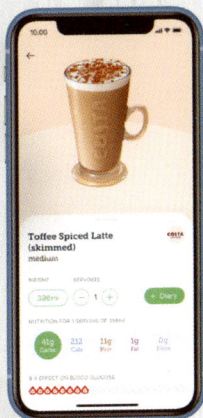 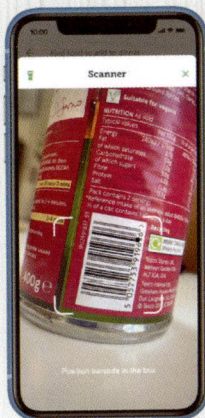 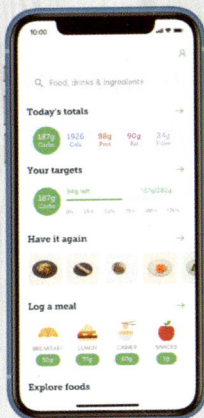 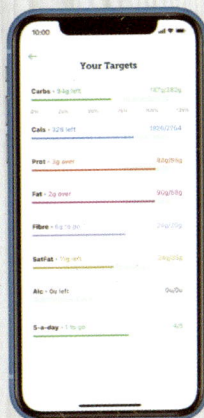

FREE 14-day trial

Download on the App Store

GET IT ON Google Play

SCAN ME for **more details!**

Contents

Introduction

Weight management can be tricky, but we're here to make it simpler for you! Consider this guide your introduction to achieving and maintaining a healthy weight. It contains easy-to-understand information with practical tips to help you achieve your personal weight goal.

In the **Healthy Weight** section, you will find recent evidence on how weight impacts health, and why this is important. You will learn about the benefits and psychology of weight loss, and guidance on physical activity.

We then delve into different **Weight Loss Methods**, such as very low calorie, intermittent fasting, low carb and intuitive eating - helping you figure out which method will be most effective for your upcoming weight loss journey.

Finally, in the **Weight Maintenance Strategies** chapter, we explore what to do after you have lost weight. This is often forgotten when thinking about weight loss, but is vital for maintaining a healthy weight in the long term.

The best part is we've done all the legwork for you. The range of Carbs & Cals BOOKS can be used with any of the suggested weight loss methods, and you can use the Carbs & Cals APP to log your meals.

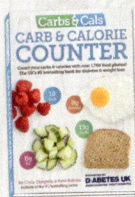

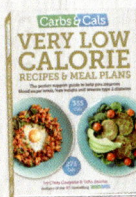

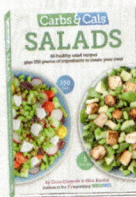

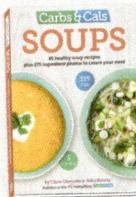

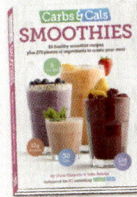

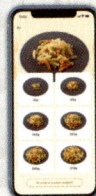

Healthy Weight

What is a healthy weight?

Everyone has a different healthy weight, which can be thought of as a weight you are able to maintain comfortably long term, that fits into your lifestyle and promotes good health.

You can check if you are currently at a healthy weight by calculating your BMI (see page 9). This is based on your weight and height, and is a useful quick check. However, one of its main limitations is that it can't distinguish between fat and muscle. You should also consider other factors such as how your clothes fit. While the number on the scales can help you keep track of your weight, it is also important to consider your overall wellbeing and lifestyle too.

A healthy weight and type 2 diabetes

Moving towards a healthier lifestyle is the primary strategy for managing type 2 diabetes. This includes achieving and maintaining a healthy weight.

If you are a healthy weight, your body is more sensitive to insulin, meaning it can use glucose from food more effectively, resulting in blood glucose levels in the healthy range.

For many people, becoming overweight reduces their body's sensitivity to insulin (known as insulin resistance), which means they are less able to use glucose from food, and their blood glucose levels are higher than normal (pre-diabetes or type 2 diabetes).

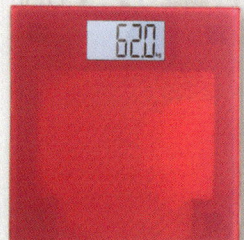

Gain Weight

Healthy Weight
Body can use insulin effectively to process glucose in food
Normal BG Levels

Overweight
Body can't use insulin properly to process glucose in food
High BG Levels (pre or type 2 diabetes)

Lose Weight

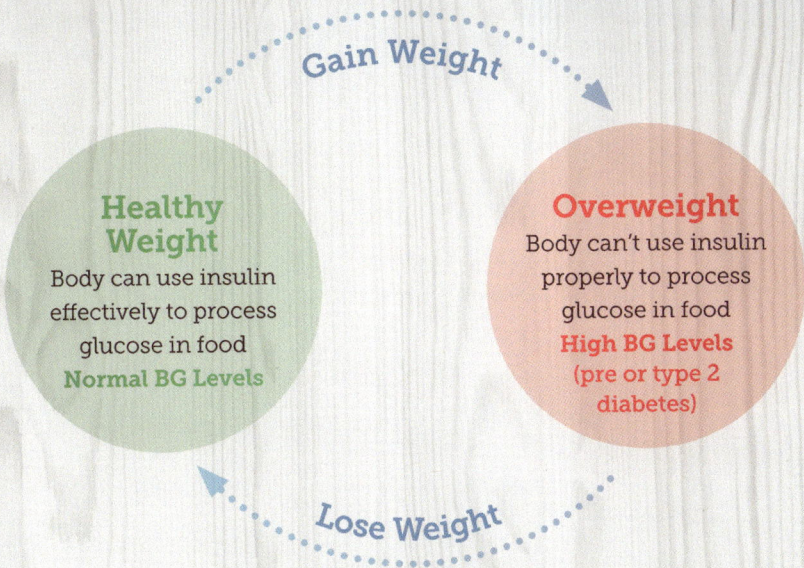

If you fall into the category on the right (overweight with high blood glucose levels), all is not lost! It's possible to put type 2 diabetes into remission (bring your blood glucose levels back down to the normal range) by losing weight and adopting a healthier lifestyle.

There are a wide range of reasons that people become overweight. Not all of these will be in your control. It is best to concentrate on areas you may be able to change and exert control over. Reasons may include:

- **Environment:** such as lifestyle and food choices, triggers to eating, and level of physical activity.

- **Medication:** Certain tablets and insulin can lead to weight gain.

- **Genetics:** Other family members may be overweight. It is important to note that this may be food choices and traditions of the family and your upbringing, and not just genetic.

- **Thyroid:** An underactive thyroid, which includes symptoms such as tiredness, weight gain, muscle weakness and sensitivity to cold. Seek advice from your GP for more information.

- **Ageing:** The older we get, the more the tendency to be less active, and our metabolism slows. Hormonal changes that occur in menopause can also be a contributing factor.

What is type 2 diabetes remission?

In recent years, it has been shown that it's possible to achieve remission from type 2 diabetes. Remission means having blood glucose levels in the healthy range (without medication), when you've previously had blood glucose levels high enough to be diagnosed with type 2 diabetes.

HbA1c Ranges		
Healthy	**Pre-diabetes**	**Type 2 diabetes**
Under 42 mmol/mol (6.0%)	42 - 47 mmol/mol (6.0 - 6.4%)	Above 48 mmol/mol (6.5%)

Recent research (the DiRECT trial) shows that for people who have had type 2 diabetes for less than 6 years, and have a BMI over 27 kg/m^2, losing more weight gives a greater chance of achieving remission of type 2 diabetes.

Weight loss	Chance of remission
10 - 15kg (1st 8lb - 2st 5lb)	6 out of 10
More than 15kg (2st 5lb)	9 out of 10

We are only just beginning to understand remission of type 2 diabetes. There is still lots to learn:

★ How long does remission last for?
★ How much weight loss is beneficial for people who have a BMI less than 27 kg/m^2?
★ What happens for people who have had type 2 diabetes for longer than 6 years?

Despite not knowing all of this, what we do know is that for most people that are overweight, any weight loss is beneficial for health.

Do I need to lose weight?

BMI

One way of knowing if you need to lose weight is by measuring your Body Mass Index (BMI). Your BMI is a measure of your weight in relation to your height, and tells you if you are a healthy weight. To work out your BMI, you can visit the online calculator at www.carbsandcals.com/BMI, ask your healthcare team, or use the following equation:

$$BMI = Weight\ (kg) \div Height\ (m)^2$$

For example, if your weight is 72kg and your height is 1.68m, then your BMI = 72 ÷ (1.68 x 1.68) = 25.5 kg/m².

Once you have your BMI, you can see which range it falls into by comparing it to this table, to see if you need to lose weight. By lowering your weight, you will lower your BMI.

BMI (kg/m²)	BMI for Black, Asian & other minority ethnic groups	Category
Under 18.5	Under 18.5	Underweight
18.5 - 24.9	**18.5 - 22.9**	**Healthy weight**
25 - 29.9	23 - 27.9	Overweight
30 or over	28 or over	Obese

People from African, Caribbean, South Asian & Chinese backgrounds are encouraged to aim for the BMI targets in the middle column above because they have 4 to 6 times more risk of developing type 2 diabetes, which develops at an earlier age. Research suggests that people from these groups are also at higher risk of conditions such as cardiovascular disease, cancer and stroke at a lower BMI, compared to people from white backgrounds.

Important note: If you have a large amount of muscle, your BMI may be in the overweight range, even though you have little body fat.

Benefits of weight loss

As already mentioned, if you have type 2 diabetes, losing weight can increase your chance of remission and bring your blood glucose levels back into the healthy range (see page 8).

If you are overweight, regardless of whether you've got type 2 diabetes or not, reducing your weight by just 5% (and maintaining that weight loss) can reduce the risk of developing:

- ★ High blood pressure
- ★ High cholesterol
- ★ Heart disease, angina and stroke
- ★ Some types of cancer
- ★ Osteoarthritis
- ★ Back and joint pain
- ★ Fertility problems

Even if you have already developed any of these health issues, weight loss can still be beneficial in improving and managing them. Losing weight is also associated with greater mobility, improved psychological health (including more positive body image) and a longer and healthier life overall.

This is what 5% weight loss looks like, depending on your starting weight:

Current weight	Weight to lose (5%)	Weight to achieve	Current weight	Weight to lose (5%)	Weight to achieve
60kg	3kg	57kg	9.5st	7lb	9st
70kg	3.5kg	66.5kg	11st	8lb	10st 6lb
80kg	4kg	76kg	12.5st	9lb	11st 12lb
90kg	4.5kg	85.5kg	14st	10lb	13st 4lb
100kg	5kg	95kg	15.5st	11lb	14st 10lb

The psychology of weight loss

A large part of your success with weight loss comes down to your own psychology: how you motivate yourself, your beliefs about yourself, how you handle "failure", and how supported you feel. To help you understand your own personal situation, consider the following questions:

> What is my motivation?

> Is now a suitable time for me to lose weight?

> What has worked for me before?

> What has not worked? How can I avoid this happening again?

> What support do I need?

> How will I reward myself for my achievements?

Our thoughts, feelings and beliefs determine our actions and behaviours. By ensuring that your thoughts, feelings and beliefs are aligned to your goals, you are more likely to achieve the required behaviours to help you get there. For example:

Belief / thought	Change to
I can't lose weight	I can lose weight and keep it off
I don't like "healthy" foods	There are some healthy foods that I enjoy and I can discover new healthy foods to enjoy
Every time I lose weight, I just put more weight back on	Losing weight and keeping it off are two different things, and I can learn to maintain my new weight

One way to think about a weight loss journey is as follows:

Not aware of a problem
You are not thinking about making any changes because you do not consider your weight a problem.

▼

Thinking about it
You are aware that your weight is affecting your health and are starting to think about making changes to change this.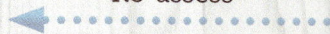

Re-assess

▼

Getting prepared
You are starting to take steps towards weight loss (e.g. reading this book, and thinking how to eat more vegetables).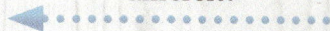

Plan something different

▼

Putting plans into action
You are taking steps to achieve weight loss (e.g. eating more vegetables at lunch time).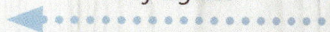

Try again

Keep doing it
You keep doing a new behaviour (e.g. you eat more vegetables at lunch time now without thinking about it).

(Adapted from the 'Stages of Change' model by Prochaska & DiClemente)

Some things to think about with this model:

Relapse
You return to your previous habits
(e.g. you have stopped eating vegetables with lunch now and eat what you used to before).

★ **Relapse is NOT a failure**
It is a normal part of changing your behaviour. The important thing is to recognise that a relapse has happened, and either try again with the same strategy, or try something different. The goal is to learn from what has happened and adapt where necessary to reduce the chances of the relapse happening again.

★ **Take your time**
Everyone moves through the stages of weight loss at a different pace. After a relapse, you may move back to any of the stages - be gentle with yourself and take time to move sustainably towards a point where you can maintain the new healthier habit. A bit like learning to drive, there will be good and not so good lessons along the way. You may not achieve your goal the first time. Keep practicing and you will inevitably get there.

★ **Get prepared**
Take your time to prepare properly. Ever heard the saying *"Prior preparation prevents pretty poor performance"*? More effort in the preparation stage leads to a greater chance of success. You would not be able to run a 10k race without putting in place a gradual training programme.

★ **Be patient**
Both time and patience are key to developing a sustainable healthier lifestyle, as it can take about 6 weeks to change a single old habit into a new behaviour.

★ **Make it manageable!**
If you take on too much too soon, you are unlikely to reach your weight loss goal and maintain it.

Changing habits

Habits are actions and behaviours that are repeated without thinking about them. When it comes to your diet, it's likely that you are on autopilot. How you eat, when you eat and your food preferences have developed over years, if not decades, and changing these habits can be tricky. Behaviours around food are ingrained in your life - this is not to say that they can't be changed, but it will take some time, effort and perseverance.

There are many ways of transforming old habits into new ones, to help you achieve your health goals. Here are some important areas to consider...

Prepare your environment

Think about the things around you. Do they support you in achieving your health goals? For example, what's in your kitchen cupboards, fridge and freezer? Do these foods make it easy for you to prepare healthy meals? If the answer is not a resounding "yes!", there may be some work to do here.

Another example: think about when you reach for that mid-morning or mid-afternoon snack. Do you automatically appear at the temptation-filled vending machine? Or is there a piece of fruit ready in your desk drawer? Consciously prepping your environment helps you make healthy eating an easier choice.

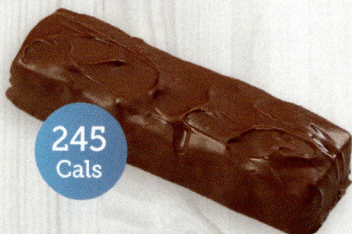

245
Cals

swap
— to →

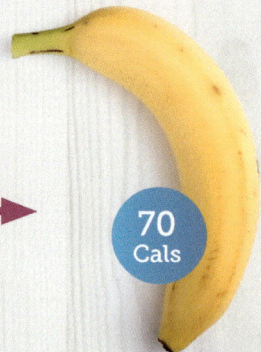

70
Cals

Address the psychology

The "why" often drives the "what" when it comes to eating. Looking at the why behind your actions will support you in making healthier choices. A common example is using calorie-dense food to soothe the stress of work and life, or to alleviate sadness. If this habit is standing in the way of you achieving your health goals, it's probably time to tackle it. Finding alternative ways to deal with these emotions (such as exercise and meditation) can help you rely less on comfort eating.

Do you eat to reward yourself? This is another common "why" that leads people to overeat. If this sounds like you, come up with a list of non-food based rewards to keep you motivated.

Start small

So small that it almost feels like it's not worth doing. The new habit may not show results any time soon, but it will allow you to build on top of it. Eventually this new habit will start showing results, at which point it is more likely to be maintained.

For example, an apple instead of a flapjack on one day of the week isn't going to shed pounds overnight, but is a realistic start for most people. Before you know it, you have developed the habit of having a piece of fruit for morning and afternoon snacks Monday to Friday (10 snacks in total) and you're consuming 1600 fewer calories over 5 days.

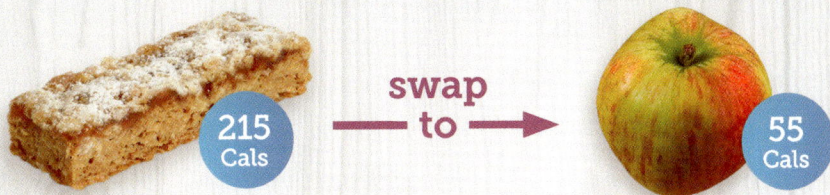

215 Cals   **swap to →**   55 Cals

Triggers to eating can come from different situations, emotions and times of the day. These can be thought of as internal such as hunger, cravings, mood changes and unhelpful thoughts, and external such as smelling food, watching others eat and seeing food, to name a few. Identifying your triggers can help you have a greater understanding of your behaviour and where to target your changes.

Dealing with slip-ups

Things are bound to go off track. When they do, use them as an opportunity to learn. Reflecting on your recent experiences and planning for the next time will help you evolve habits that work and are more sustainable long term. For example:

What happened?

I went out to eat with colleagues after work and I did not order a healthier meal as I had planned to do

▼

Why did it happened?

| My colleagues encouraged me to make an unhealthy choice | The healthy choice I selected was not available | After a stressful day at work, I felt like I deserved a treat |

▼

Does this happen often?

| **No** | **Yes** |
| It only happens once every 2 months, so I can focus on other habits that need changing | I eat with colleagues twice a week |

▼

Problem solving *(think of as many solutions as possible)*

| I will talk to colleagues before I go to explain that I am trying to make healthier food choices, which is very important to me, and I would appreciate their support when I'm doing this | When looking at the menu, I will choose 2 or 3 healthy options, in case one is not available | I am going to explore different ways to treat myself that do not include food, and also think about ways of managing stress at work |

Remember, nobody is 100% motivated 100% of the time. Motivation, willpower and enthusiasm rise and fall depending on a number of factors. Persevere and accept that you may slip up from time to time. Do everything in your ability to stay on track as much as possible, and don't beat yourself up when it doesn't go as planned. Practise self-compassion and patience, build resilience and be flexible to adapt where necessary.

Top Tips for getting back on track

- **GET SUPPORT** from a friend or family member who can act as an accountability partner. If you do go off track, talk to them about why it happened and your ideas for problem solving.

- **KEEP A JOURNAL** of your success. That way when slip-ups happen you can look back and see your success written down.

- **REMEMBER** that a few slip-ups will not derail your overall success. Your journey to changing long term behaviour is supposed to have twists and turns. Slip-ups are a great way to learn more about yourself.

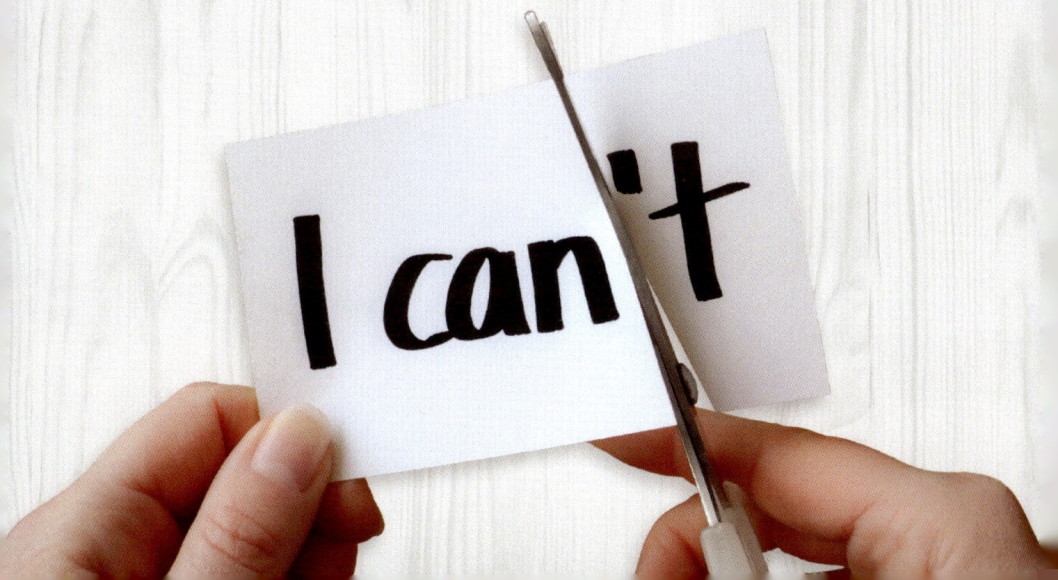

Eating out, special events & holidays

Any event that breaks away from your usual routine is a great opportunity to practise your weight management skills. Explore new lower calorie foods, cuisines, cooking techniques and drinks that align with your diet objectives.

Top tips for eating away from home

★ Look at the restaurant menu online (or check the Carbs & Cals APP) the day before, so you can plan the rest of your day in advance. You may change your usual lunch option if you know what you'll be eating at the restaurant.

★ Don't starve yourself before you eat out, as you are more likely to overeat on high calorie foods. Frequent meals also support more stable blood glucose levels.

★ Ask the people around you to support and encourage you in your food choices. You may discuss this with them in advance of going out, so it's not a surprise.

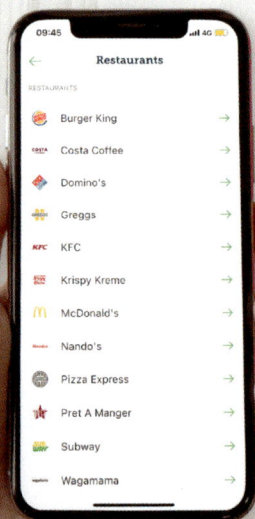

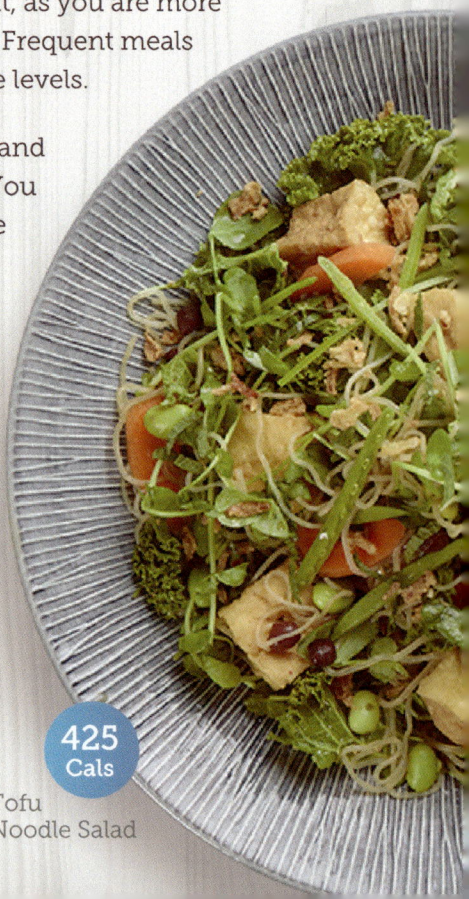

425 Cals

Tofu Noodle Salad

09:45

Restaurants

RESTAURANTS

Burger King →
Costa Coffee →
Domino's →
Greggs →
KFC →
Krispy Kreme →
McDonald's →
Nando's →
Pizza Express →
Pret A Manger →
Subway →
Wagamama →

★ A great way to keep calories down is to opt out of starters and/or desserts. Or why not share? That way, you still get to try the yummy food, but with half the calories.

★ Remember to think about what you drink! These are often forgotten about and can add up to a hefty amount of calories (sometimes more than the meal). Also keep in mind that an increase in alcohol can lead to a decrease in healthy food choices!

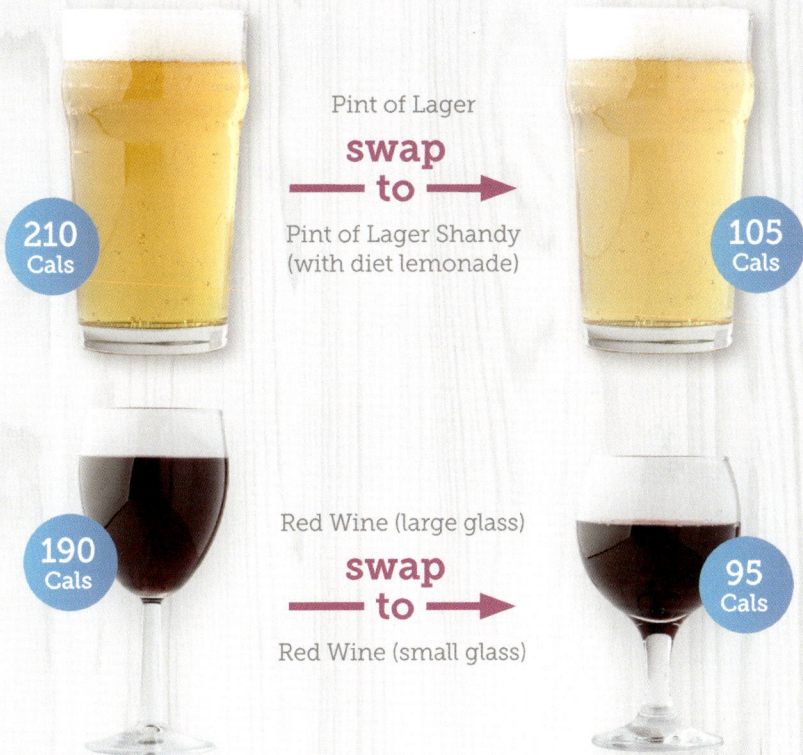

Pint of Lager

swap to →

210 Cals

105 Cals

Red Wine (large glass)

swap to →

Red Wine (small glass)

190 Cals

95 Cals

★ If you eat something you didn't plan to, don't beat yourself up - enjoy it! All food can be part of a healthy lifestyle, and there is no shame in eating any food.

★ Special events often centre around food and drink, but remember there are other ways to mark an occasion. For example, you could plan an outdoor walk, a game in the park or a painting class, rather than going out to solely focus on eating and drinking.

Support networks

Don't feel you need to do everything on your own. You are going to need help on the path to successfully changing your behaviours. Without the support, you may be tempted to give up, especially during the times you feel unmotivated, frustrated or incapable.

Identifying the type of support you need and where you can get it from means that you are more likely to achieve success in behaviour change. The diagram below is an example of how you can map out your support system. Having lots of different sources of help means you get a well balanced support system that you can call on when needed.

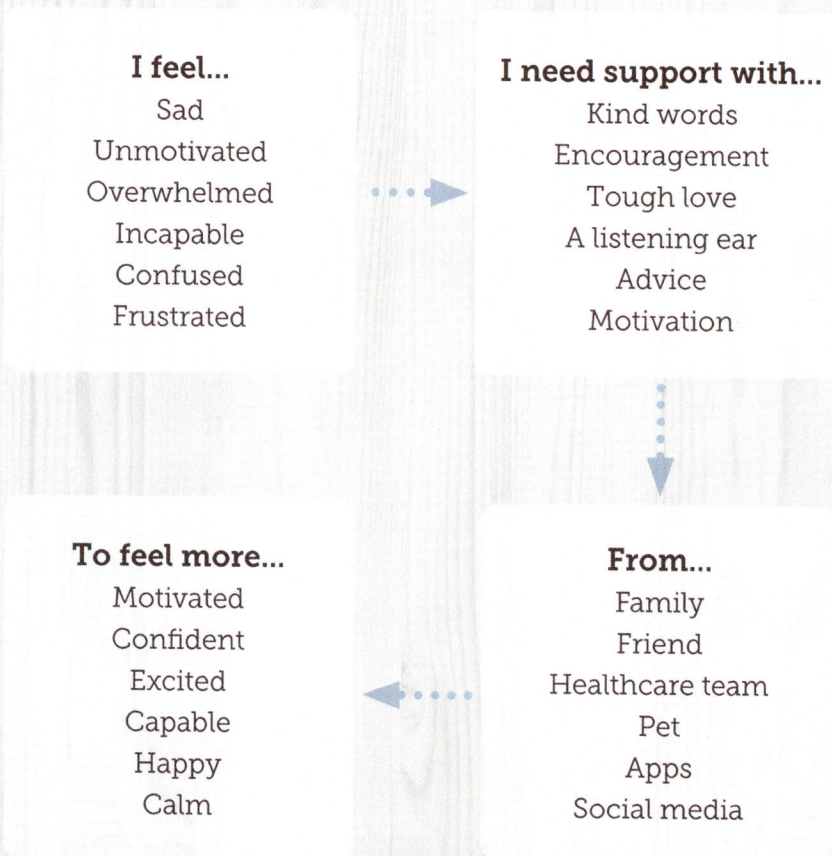

I feel...
Sad
Unmotivated
Overwhelmed
Incapable
Confused
Frustrated

I need support with...
Kind words
Encouragement
Tough love
A listening ear
Advice
Motivation

To feel more...
Motivated
Confident
Excited
Capable
Happy
Calm

From...
Family
Friend
Healthcare team
Pet
Apps
Social media

Sleep

Sleep is an essential component of health and wellbeing, allowing us to rest and recover from the physical and mental activity we experience throughout the day. An average adult requires 7 to 9 hours of sleep each night, and if you have less than this there is an increased risk of health issues, such as heart disease and stress. Stress hormones increase insulin resistance, so if you have type 2 diabetes, ensuring you get regular quality sleep can help with this. Additionally, getting enough sleep and minimising stress also means you have more mental strength to stick to your weight loss plan.

Sleep is impacted by many factors including diet, exercise, environment, mental state and routine. If you aren't sleeping well at the moment, take some time to notice what happened during the day that may have contributed to the restless night. The goal is to identify specific factors that have stopped you from sleeping well, so you can alter these where possible.

For example, did you eat particularly sugary or salty foods (like a takeaway or processed food) in the evening? Do you tend to sleep poorly after drinking alcohol? Was the environment too hot or bright? Perhaps a thinner duvet or sleep mask could be simple solutions.

Consider some sleep hygiene principles like reducing caffeine intake, practising mindfulness before bed, going to sleep and waking up at a similar time each day, and no screen time 1 hour before bed. Charge your phone overnight in a different room to avoid night-time phone disturbance and temptation. Use an alarm clock instead of your phone if you need a wakeup call.

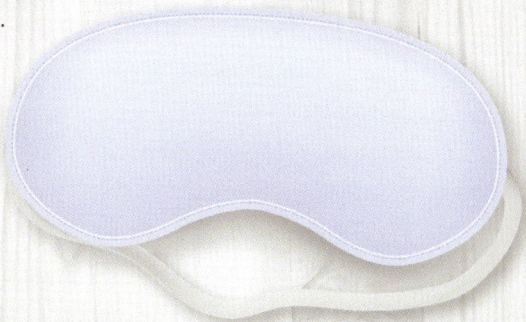

Physical activity

There are many benefits to physical activity and there is strong evidence to show that regular activity can reduce the risks of major illnesses, such as:

Heart disease & stroke

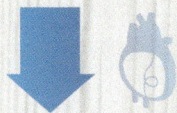

35%

Cancers

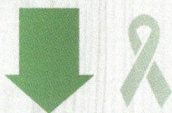

20-50%

Falls

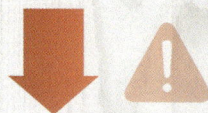

30%

Osteoarthritis

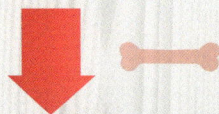

83%

Depression & dementia

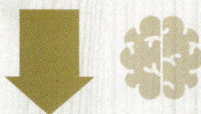

30%

Early death

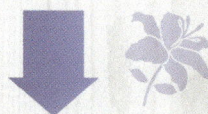

30%

If you have type 2 diabetes, physical activity can also make you more insulin sensitive. Engaging in regular physical activity will not only support healthy weight management, it may mean using less medication for type 2 diabetes.

One of the great things about physical activity is that it works for all ages, sizes and abilities. You can personalise activity to your ability and level - it's all about doing more than you currently do. You don't need fancy equipment, expensive gym memberships or a lot of time. Something as simple as breaking sedentary behaviour by standing up occasionally, a 5 minute walk or a 10 minute chair-based set of exercises are great ways to start.

The current physical activity guidelines for healthy adults are:

Option 1	Option 2	Option 3
At least **150 mins** of **moderate intensity exercise** (increased breathing but able to talk) per week	At least **75 mins** of **vigorous intensity activity** (breathing fast and difficult to talk) per week	A mixture of Option **1** and Option **2**

AND weight bearing exercise (bodyweight or other weights) on 2 days of the week

For older adults (over 65 years), also consider activities that **improve balance** on 2 days of the week

If you have diabetes and are taking insulin or certain tablets that lower blood glucose, talk to your healthcare team if you start to increase your level of physical activity significantly, as you may need to adjust medication.

This is because you will be using up more glucose for energy and your body becomes more sensitive to the insulin. The likelihood of a low blood glucose level (hypo) can increase if you don't make adjustments to medication. You may also be asked to check your blood glucose level more frequently by your healthcare team.

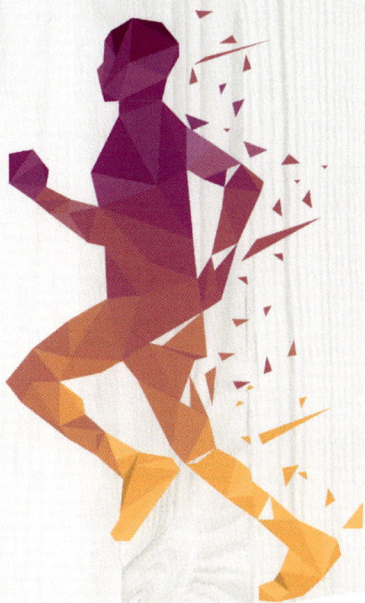

Weight Loss Methods

Weight loss is about using up more calories than you take in. This is called a calorie deficit. General guidance is that a 500 calorie deficit every day achieves a weight loss of about ¼ to ½ kg (½ to 1 lb) per week. This will depend on the individual and the point in their weight loss journey. The greater the deficit, the faster the weight loss.

This calorie deficit can be achieved in a variety of ways, and different methods suit different people. Some people may choose to increase their activity levels to use up more calories, but keep their food intake the same. Others change the food they eat to reduce calories going in, but keep physical activity the same. Many people make small changes to both their food and physical activity, to achieve the calorie deficit from both angles.

Research shows that no single diet is universally most effective for everyone. For example, some people find that a low carb approach works for them, and others achieve results more easily using the very low calorie diet. Choosing a way of eating that suits you, your environment and social situation is more likely to achieve long term weight loss. Whichever path you select, having the skills, knowledge and support is key.

There are various methods of losing weight. Here we explore some of the more common methods, which are grounded in scientific research and evidence.

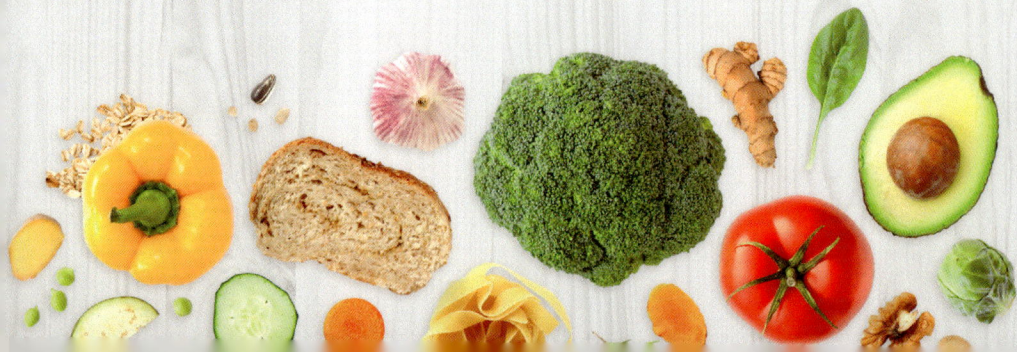

What is a calorie?

All food and drinks contain energy. Just like we measure length in metres or feet, we measure energy in calories. Some nutrients give more energy than others:

1g carbohydrate = 4 cals

1g protein = 4 cals

1g fat = 9 cals

1g alcohol = 7 cals

Our body uses energy (or calories) in 3 main ways:
- ★ Keeping us ticking over
  (e.g. keeping our heart beating and immune system healthy)
- ★ Digesting food
- ★ All daily activities (e.g. walking, working or going for a run)

If you eat and drink the **same** amount of calories as your body needs, your weight will **stay the same**

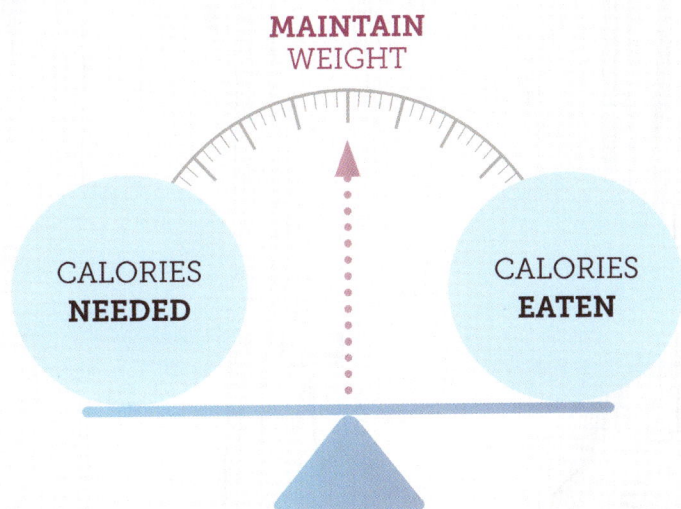

MAINTAIN
WEIGHT

CALORIES
NEEDED

CALORIES
EATEN

If you eat and drink **more** calories than your body needs, the extra energy is stored as fat and you **gain weight**

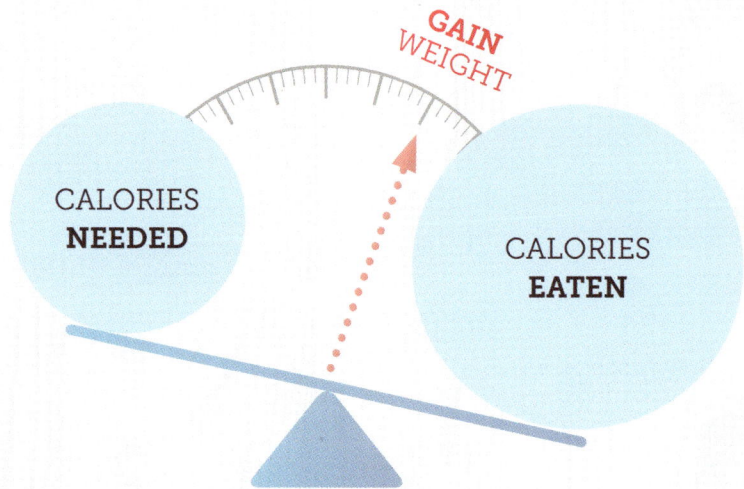

GAIN
WEIGHT

CALORIES
NEEDED

CALORIES
EATEN

If you eat and drink **less** calories than your body needs, you will use up fat stores and **lose weight**

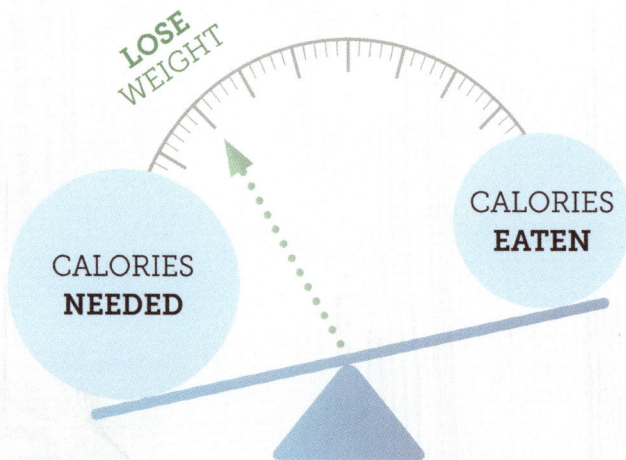

LOSE
WEIGHT

CALORIES
NEEDED

CALORIES
EATEN

Another consideration is that not all calories have the same nutritional benefit and impact on the body. A handful of chewy sweets and a large banana both contain around 100 calories.

★ The chewy sweets are made of processed sugar (with no other nutrients) and therefore cause a rapid change in blood glucose levels (high glycaemic index or GI).

★ On the other hand, the banana is a mixture of starchy carbs and natural sugars. It contains vitamins, minerals and fibre, and causes a more gradual change to blood glucose levels (medium GI).

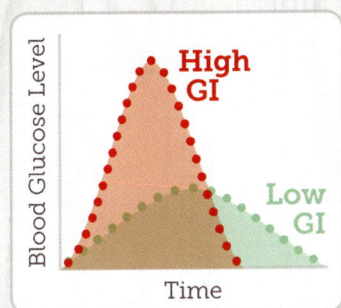

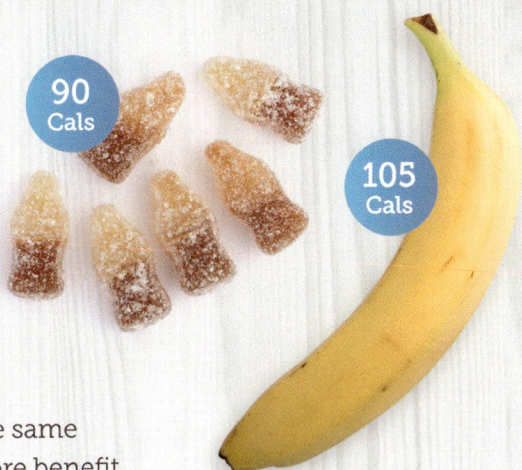

Even though both foods have the same calories, nutritionally there is more benefit of eating a banana than chewy sweets.

There is also research to suggest that some of the calories in high fibre foods are used by our gut bacteria, leaving fewer calories to cause weight gain. The Carbs & Cals SALADS & SOUPS recipe books have lots of high fibre recipe ideas.

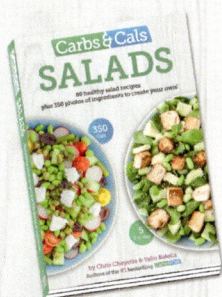

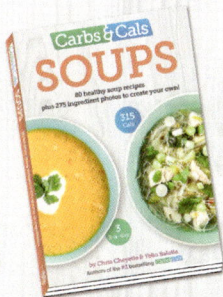

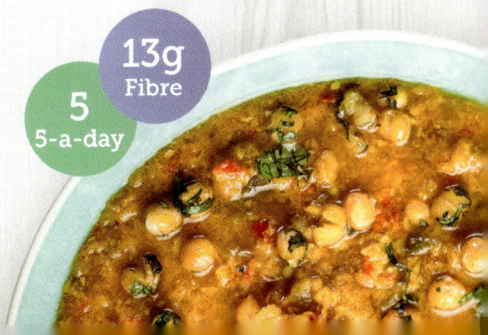

How many calories do I need?

For weight maintenance, the average man requires approximately 2500 calories per day, and the average woman needs around 2000 calories. However, these are just averages and your specific calorie requirements are based on your weight, height, age and activity level.

There's an easy way to work out how many calories you need, using the Carbs & Cals calorie requirement calculator:

www.carbsandcals.com/BMI

You can use the handy tool to discover how many calories you personally need to maintain weight. Once you know this, you can choose a weight loss method that results in a calorie deficit.

Calorie controlled diet

A calorie controlled diet is where you eat a specific amount of calories each day to achieve a calorie deficit and lose weight. For example, this could be 1800, 1500 or 1200 calories per day.

Making any reduction in your usual calorie intake is a great start, to work towards your new calorie target. Changing some of the foods you eat, altering cooking methods, and reducing portion sizes can all add up to make a difference in your daily calorie consumption.

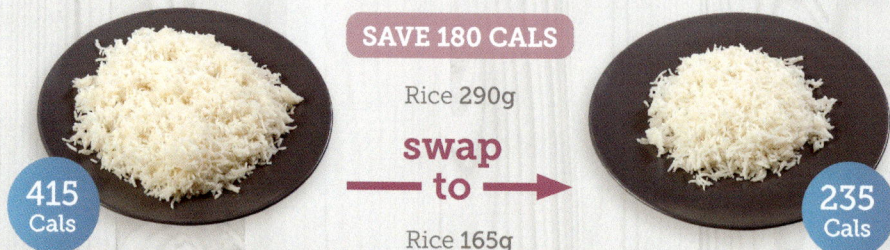

SAVE 180 CALS

Rice 290g

swap to →

Rice 165g

415 Cals

235 Cals

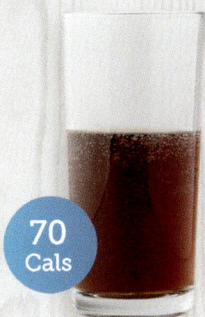
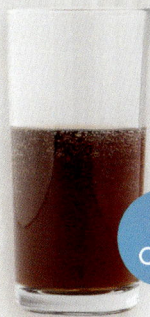

SAVE 70 CALS

Cola 165ml
(half a can)

swap to →

Diet Cola 165ml
(half a can)

70 Cals

0 Cals

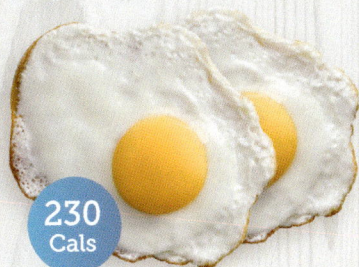
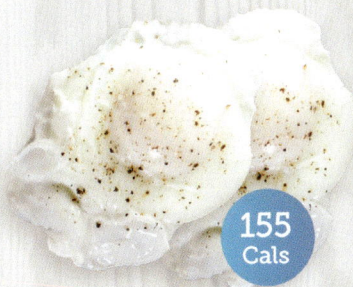

SAVE 75 CALS

2 Fried Eggs

swap to →

2 Poached Eggs

230 Cals

155 Cals

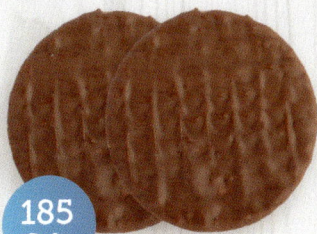
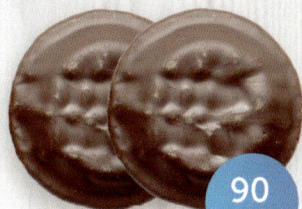

SAVE 95 CALS

2 Chocolate
Oat Biscuits

swap to →

2 Jaffa Cakes

185 Cals

90 Cals

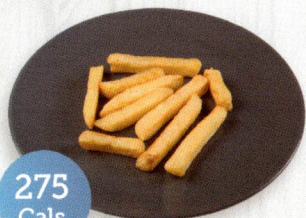
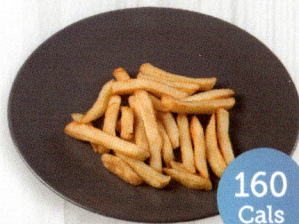

SAVE 115 CALS

Deep Fried Chips 100g

swap to →

Oven Chips 100g

275 Cals

160 Cals

Let's look at an example day and see how we can make swaps to achieve a 500 calorie reduction.

If you usually eat...

	Foods	Cals	5-a-day
Breakfast	Porridge (whole milk), 1 tbsp peanut butter, handful blueberries	340	½
Snack	Latte (whole milk), 30g almonds	320	0
Lunch	BLT sandwich, crisps, apple, 250ml orange juice	725	2¾
Snack	Chocolate wafer bar	105	0
Dinner	Chicken & noodle stir-fry, fruit yogurt pot	535	2
After Dinner	Large glass of white wine, sweet popcorn	290	0
Daily Totals		**2315**	**5¼**

To save 500 calories, swap to...

	Foods	Cals	5-a-day
Breakfast	Porridge (semi-skimmed milk), 1 tbsp peanut butter, handful blueberries	290 **SAVE 50 CALS**	½
Snack	Flat white (skimmed milk), 15g almonds, satsuma	195 **SAVE 125 CALS**	1
Lunch	Chicken salad sandwich, houmous & dippers, babybel light, apple, water	540 **SAVE 185 CALS**	2¼
Snack	Chocolate wafer bar	105	0
Dinner	Smaller portion chicken & noodle stir-fry with mangetout, fruit yogurt pot	480 **SAVE 55 CALS**	2½
After Dinner	Small glass of white wine, salted popcorn	190 **SAVE 100 CALS**	0
Daily Totals		1800	6¼

The new meal plan saves 500 calories and still includes chocolate, wine, popcorn and more than 5 portions of fruit and veg. This shows how little swaps throughout the day can add up to achieve the 500 calorie reduction. The Carbs & Cals APP is a quick and easy way to check and track the calorie values of all the food you eat.

You may find the changes suggested here are too much, or you may feel like you can do more. If you aim for fewer calories (e.g. 1200) per day, you will lose weight more quickly, and if your target is higher (e.g. 1800 calories), you will lose weight more slowly - as long as you don't go over the number of calories needed for weight maintenance, of course!

To get used to eating fewer calories, you may for example choose to start with an 1800 calorie meal plan for a few weeks, then move to one with 1500 calories. There is no fixed way of doing this, so take your time and experiment to find a strategy that works for you.

It is important to be aware that there is a limit to how much you should reduce your calorie intake. Always consult a medical professional before making any big changes, especially if you have a medical condition or are taking regular medications. You should also not aim for weight loss during pregnancy.

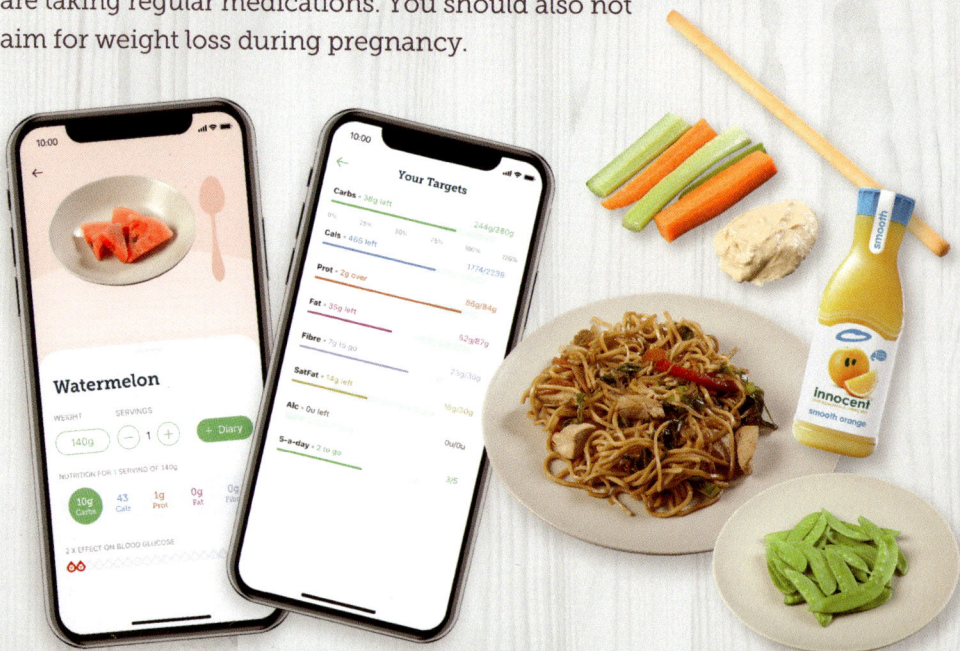

Very low calorie diet

A very low calorie diet (VLCD) is defined as eating up to 800 calories a day. This is a really low amount of calories, and should be carried out with support and supervision (especially if you have health conditions, such as diabetes). VLCD can offer rapid and dramatic weight loss, and can be followed safely for a maximum of 3 months. It can be done with meal replacements or with food.

Before embarking on a VLCD, there are some initial side effects to consider, such as headaches, nausea, constipation (more so with the meal replacement method), fatigue and bad breath. However, it is an effective approach and can kickstart your weight loss journey, as you may find it very motivating to see yourself losing weight rapidly.

Completion of the VLCD (maximum of 3 months) is usually followed by a gradual increase in calories, often going onto a different weight loss or weight maintenance plan.

This might include gradually adding back in one meal a day if you are using meal replacement drinks. Or increasing the calories of your meals by having more carbs or larger portions if you are using a food based approach.

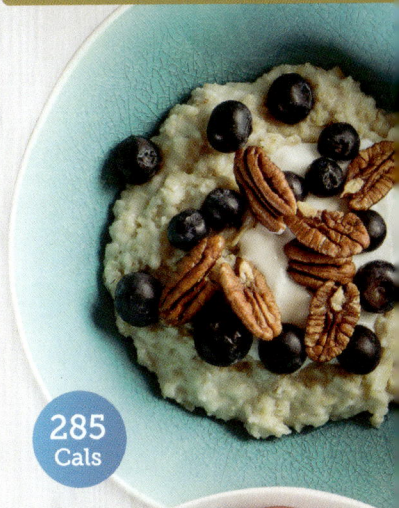

285
Cals

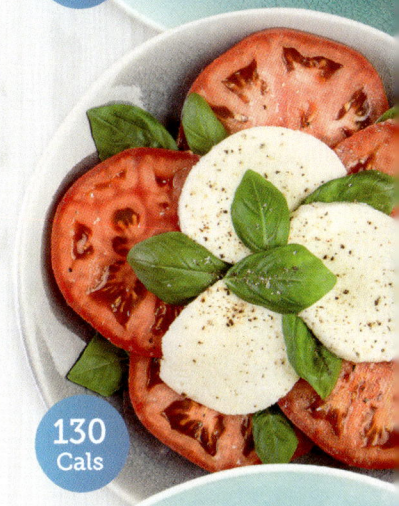

130
Cals

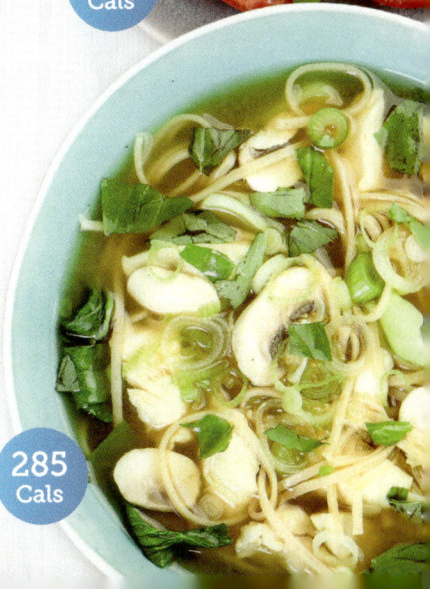

285
Cals

Meal replacement VLCD

This method uses specialist supplements (soups, shakes & bars) to provide a nutritionally complete diet. The benefit of using supplements is that it takes less thought, planning and time preparing food each day. People tend to find this easy to follow.

Companies offering these supplements include 1:1 by the Cambridge Diet Plan, Lighter Life, Exante, and Shake that Weight (for women). These typically involve 3 or 4 shakes, soups or bars per day (instead of meals) for 12 weeks, so perhaps a shake at breakfast, bar at lunch and soup at dinner making a total of 600 to 800 calories.

The next stage is a gradual reintroduction of foods, aiming for a higher calorie intake (e.g. 1200 calories) by eating a healthy meal and snack each day, with 2 or 3 of the supplement products.

One advantage of this approach is that it takes away the need for planning out all your meals and for food preparation. This can be an attractive prospect for some people.

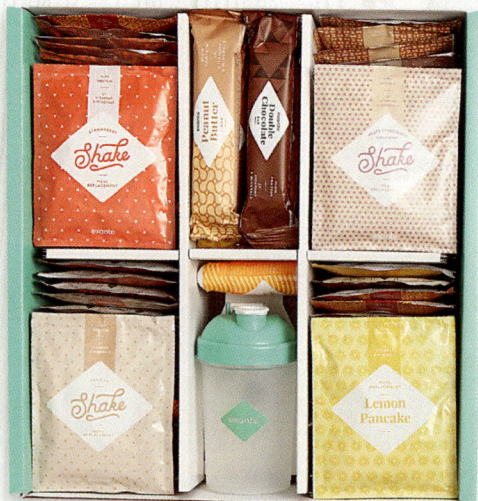

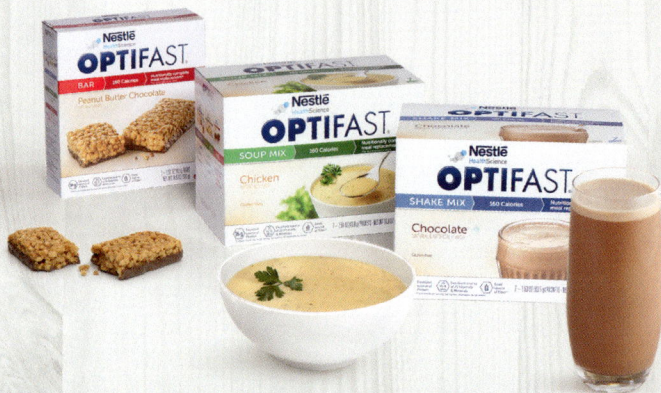

Food based VLCD

This method allows you to still eat whole food and is great if you wish to keep some of your usual foods in your diet. You can use the Carbs & Cals VERY LOW CALORIE RECIPES & MEAL PLANS book to help you plan nutritious and delicious meals. This book guides you through meals and snacks to get to a total of around 800 calories a day, and has a wealth of options to keep it interesting, satisfying and tasty. How does avocado and eggs for breakfast, steak and olive salad for lunch, and Jamaican chicken curry for dinner sound?

It's worth thinking about which approach will suit you. Having foods can feel more normal, offer variability and be more sociable, but it does take more prep - both in terms of food shopping and planning. You will also need to make sure you control portions carefully, otherwise you might be going to all this effort, yet eating more than you realise. All the recipes in the Carbs & Cals VERY LOW CALORIE RECIPES & MEAL PLANS book are weighed out, so you know you're staying on track.

215 Cals

225 Cals

270 Cals

360 Cals

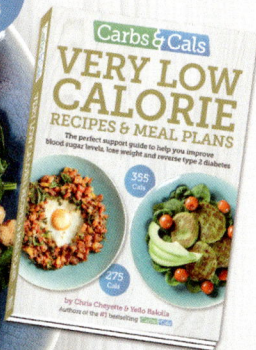

Intermittent fasting

Intermittent fasting is a relatively new approach to weight management with an increasing amount of research to support it. Like the diets already discussed, the aim is to reduce your overall calorie intake. The difference with this method is that it focuses on restricting calorie intake only during a specific period of time. This could mean only limiting calories 2 days per week (i.e. the 5:2 diet), or fasting completely for a set number of hours each day (e.g. the 16:8 diet). Both methods have the overall effect of reducing your average weekly calorie intake - helping you to lose weight.

The main advantage of intermittent fasting is that you are not dieting all of the time. It enables you to lose weight without the feeling of constant deprivation. With food restrictions implemented only some of the time, you can achieve a significant reduction in overall calories, whilst being flexible with food choices the rest of the time.

Some people find that this style of eating fits in with their life, and provides structure and routine without too much planning. There are quite a few types of intermittent fasting patterns, but here we focus on the two more mainstream versions: the 5:2 and 16:8.

5:2

The 5:2 diet reduces your weekly calorie intake by 25%, while requiring you to diet for only 2 days a week. You eat a normal healthy diet 5 days a week, and fast on the remaining 2 days. You can change your 2 fasting days each week to fit in with your schedule and social engagements. This has proven to be an effective method for many people.

Instead of feeling restricted every day, you focus on just 2 days of the week (which can be consecutive or non consecutive). On these 2 days, you eat a very low number of calories: 500 for a woman and 600 for a man.

On fasting days, you can experiment with how to structure the day to manage hunger and energy levels. Sometimes it takes a few fasting days to work out the most suitable plan for you. There are a number of ways you can achieve your calorie target. This might be 2 x 250 calorie meals, or even 5 x 100 calorie meals / snacks throughout the day if 3 meal times doesn't work for you.

Here are a few examples of how you might break up a daily 500 calorie allowance:

Scenario	Meal Structure
If you are in a rush in the morning with little time to prepare breakfast, it may be easier for you to skip breakfast and have:	Lunch: **250 cals** Dinner: **250 cals**
Busy at work through the day? Try missing lunch:	Breakfast: **250 cals** Dinner: **250 cals**
If you prefer the idea of 3 meals a day, have 3 smaller meals:	Breakfast: **150 cals** Lunch: **150 cals** Dinner: **200 cals**
Some people find that eating little and often works best to help keep hunger away through the day:	Breakfast: **100 cals** Mid-morning Snack: **50 cals** Lunch: **100 cals** Afternoon Snack: **50 cals** Dinner: **200 cals**

When starting the 5:2 diet, fasting days aren't always easy, and you may find doing them on busy days can offer some welcomed distraction from thinking about food. Other tips include making sure that you're drinking enough calorie free drinks like water, herbal teas, sugar free squash and fizzy water, aiming for at least 2 litres. Also, try to choose foods and snacks that are higher in protein as this will help to keep you feeling full and satisfied.

On the other 5 days, it's recommended that you eat a healthy balanced diet with the occasional treat, rather than bingeing, and these might be the days you feel more comfortable to include physical activity.

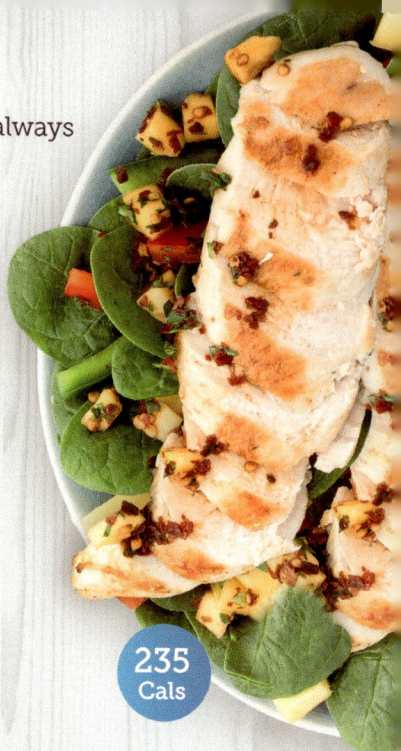

235 Cals

Example 500 calorie meal plan:

Dish	Cals	Prot	Fibre	5-a-day
Tofu Scramble	135	13g	3g	2
Tomato & Red Pepper Soup	110	3g	5g	2½
Okra & Lentil Curry	255	14g	12g	4
Totals	500	30g	20g	8½

16:8

Where the 5:2 is referring to non-fasting and fasting *days*, the 16:8 refers to *hours* of fasting and non-fasting each day. Strict timings and structure (which really appeal to some people) are key to the success of this weight loss method.

The first number is the number of consecutive hours in a 24 hour period where you don't consume any calories (i.e. the 16 hour fasting period). The second number is the remaining hours in the cycle that you can eat and drink (i.e. the 8 hour eating window).

The 8 hour eating window can be at any time you choose. For example, you can eat between 10am and 6pm (8 hours), and then fast from 6pm until 10am the following day (16 hours). This may mean moving your day around a little: perhaps a later breakfast and an earlier evening meal.

If you're someone who tends to graze in the evenings, the 16:8 could be a challenging diet to get used to, but could also be really effective to set some healthier evening habits. If you are new to dieting, the 16:8 is a great place to start, as it's extremely easy to follow and can fit into a wide variety of lifestyles.

As with the 5:2 diet, it is important to note that the 8 hour eating window is not meant to be a time to eat anything and everything. Healthy eating principles still apply and you should aim to eat a wide range of foods from all food groups.

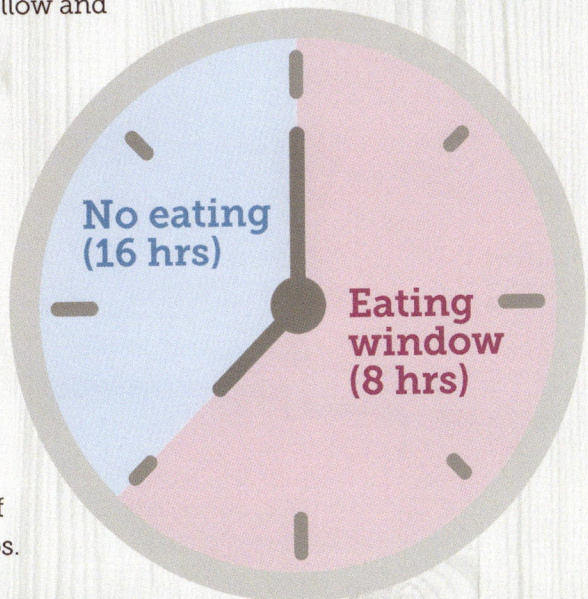

No eating
(16 hrs)

Eating
window
(8 hrs)

Low carb diet

There is no strict definition for a low carb diet. However, low carb is generally accepted as consuming between 50g and 130g carbs per day, and a *very* low carb diet can be thought of as less than 50g carbs per day.

Type of diet	Carbs per day
Typical carb intake	130g to 250g
Low carb	50g to 130g
Very low carb	Under 50g

This approach allows you to focus on reducing just one food group: carbs. Having this simple focus can be an attractive idea to some people. Done properly, this method can be effective for weight loss, especially for people with type 2 diabetes. Because carbohydrate is the nutrient that has the biggest effect on blood glucose, a low carb diet also helps to regulate and lower blood glucose levels.

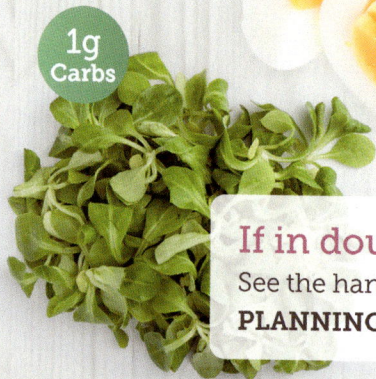

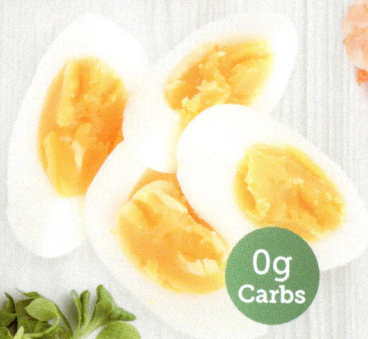

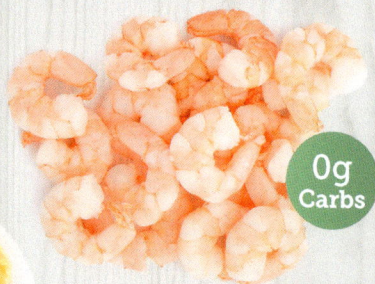

0g Carbs

1g Carbs

0g Carbs

Carbs & Cals
MEAL PLANNING GUIDE

If in doubt, check the label!

See the handy **Carbs & Cals MEAL PLANNING GUIDE** for some top tips.

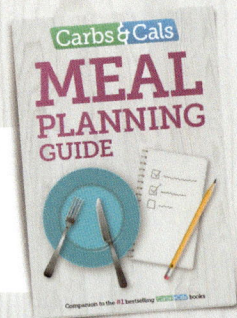

Before starting a low carb diet, it's essential to know which foods contain carbohydrate. Carbs can be found in bread, pasta, rice, potatoes, grains, cereal, lentils, beans, fruit and anything made with flour. Milk and yogurt also contain carbs in the form of lactose, and another type of carbs is sugar, which is found in fruit juices, smoothies, sweets, biscuits, cakes, honey, table sugar and jam.

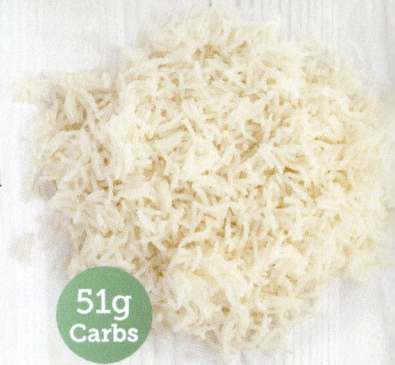

51g Carbs

A great place to start is focusing on replacing carb-dense foods with more vegetables and salad foods (excluding potato, cassava, plantain etc, which contain a lot of carbs).

12g Carbs

When you reduce carbs, be conscious of what you might be replacing them with. If you swap the carbs for foods high in fat and saturated fat, you may be inadvertently increasing unhealthy fats and risk of cardiovascular disease.

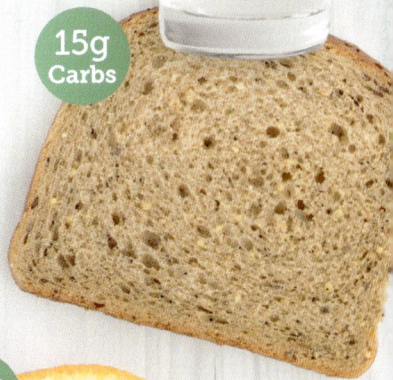

15g Carbs

It is still unclear if a low carb diet reduces weight because of a calorie deficit or it is due to other factors. To ensure weight loss on a low carb diet, consume a lower amount of calories than you eat currently.

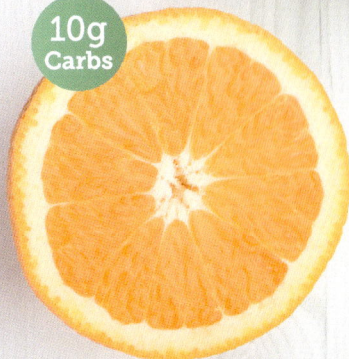

10g Carbs

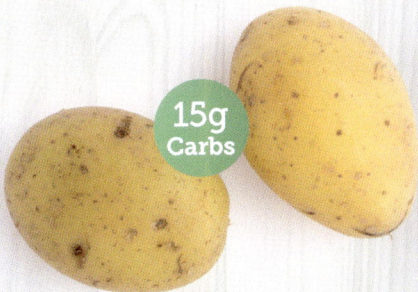

15g Carbs

Example day under 130g carbs

Breakfast	2 slices of medium granary toast with 2 poached eggs & spinach		30g carbs
Lunch	Dill Salmon & Potato Salad		26g carbs
Dinner	Quinoa, Chickpea & Spinach Soup		42g carbs
Snack	Black Forest Fruit & Mixed Seed Smoothie		25g carbs
		Total	**123g carbs**

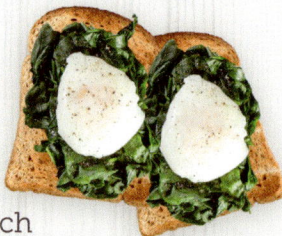

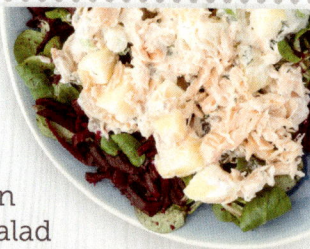

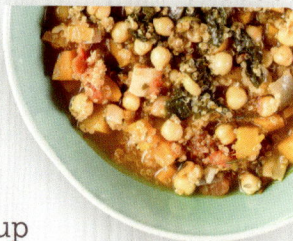

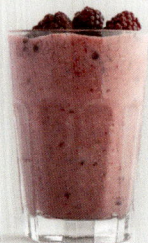

Top tips for following a low carb diet:

★ It's easy to accidentally dish out a larger portion of carb foods (e.g. rice or pasta) than you may think, so weigh out the portion of carb rich foods to make sure you're having your chosen amount. You can even weigh out the correct amount of raw rice or pasta, so you don't cook (and eat!) more than you need.

★ Fill up on veg and lean sources of protein, such as skinless chicken or fish.

★ Choose high fibre, wholegrain carbs (such as wholemeal bread, oats, brown rice and whole wheat pasta), which will help you feel fuller for longer.

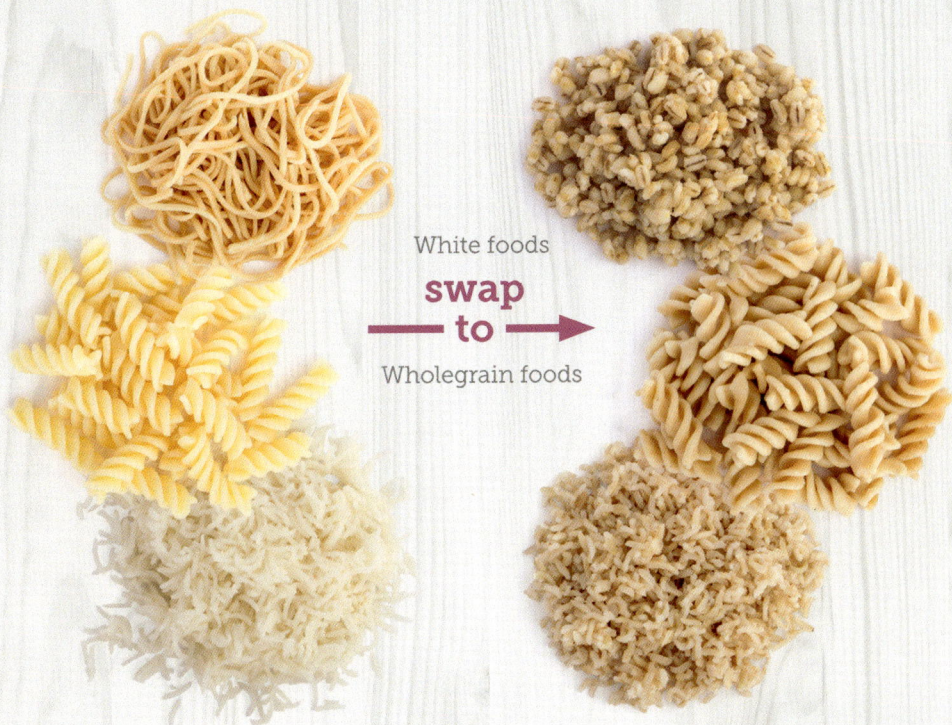

White foods

swap
to →

Wholegrain foods

If you have diabetes that is managed with tablets or insulin, it is recommended to consult your healthcare team before starting a low carb diet, as your medication may need adjusting.

Intuitive eating

Intuitive eating is a way of eating by following 10 simple guidelines. It is not intended to be used for weight loss, but more to have a healthier relationship with food. However, intuitive eating can help to implement a different mindset, leading to changes in healthy eating habits, weight loss and positive impacts on type 2 diabetes too.

The 10 rules for intuitive eating are:

1 **Reject the fad diet mentality**
Fad diets don't work, so this is a move to change your way of eating in the long term.

2 **Make peace with food**
Give yourself freedom rather than restrictions, and trust your instincts, knowing you are able to enjoy a range of foods in a balanced way.

3 **Challenge the food police**
No food is inherently "good" or "bad".

4 **Honour your hunger**
It's ok to feel hungry for food!

5 **Discover the satisfaction factor**
Be aware and recognise that you can enjoy foods and be satisfied without going overboard.

6 Feel your fullness

Eating past the point of fullness can easily happen, so practise mindful eating by listening to your body and recognise when you are full.

7 Cope with your emotions without using food

It is natural for food to comfort us, but it is not the only tool. Explore soothing music, distracting puzzles or seek a friendly hug.

8 Respect your body

Acknowledge all the wonderful things your body does and be grateful for how marvellous it is!

9 Move

Movement and exercise are a thing of joy, not punishment. Think about the ways you enjoy being active, and get moving your body!

10 Be aware

Knowing the proportions of foods to enjoy in your diet and understanding food labels will help guide you towards healthier choices.

Which diet do I choose?

There are many styles of eating and different diets available, which provide potential options for weight loss. These can be prompted by a specific health condition, ethical considerations, or may just be what the latest Hollywood superstar is promoting!

On one hand, this is great because it gives you more options. On the other hand, some of these promoted methods are not based on scientific evidence - these are known as 'fad diets'. Because fad diets aren't based on research, there is a danger they may not be healthy, and for this reason it's wise to avoid them.

To help you distinguish a healthy diet from a faddy one, ask yourself the following questions:

- ★ Does this diet promote drastic weight loss quickly?

- ★ Is this diet short term?

- ★ Is it very restrictive to a few foods, or a combination of foods?

- ★ Does it have a high price tag?

- ★ Is there a lack of credible and unbiased evidence?

- ★ Does it have special or magical ingredients?

If you answer yes to one or more of these questions, you may be looking at a fad diet!

Whatever path you choose, be mindful that eliminating entire food groups means that you may be missing out on vital nutrition. If you are unsure, or would like a professional unbiased opinion, it is worth checking with a dietitian to discuss which diet is going to be most effective for you.

TASK: Thinking about what you are hoping to achieve in the next 6 months, take a few minutes to consider the following questions:

My goal is...

I want to achieve this because...

I will need to do the following to achieve my goal...

Weight Maintenance Strategies

You've reached your target weight? Firstly, well done on your effort, as you've probably made many changes over the past few weeks, months (or years)! Achieving your target weight is the first stage of the weight loss journey, but the next stage (and arguably the more difficult) is maintaining your weight. You will have picked up valuable skills along the way that you can apply in this next phase, to help keep you around your target weight.

Weight maintenance (keeping the same weight) means that you use up the same amount of calories as you take in (see diagram on page 25). Remember, now that you are a lower weight, you will need fewer calories as there is less of you! You can use the BMI & Calorie Requirement Calculator on the Carbs & Cals website to work out the number of calories to aim for each day, to keep your weight the same. Visit www.carbsandcals.com/BMI and select the "maintain weight" option.

Fluctuations are normal, and to be expected. Weight maintenance does not mean keeping that number on the scales exactly the same, and there'll be days where clothes seem tighter or baggier than others. If you notice the number on the scales going up consistently, don't panic. Think about the following:

★ Has my routine changed?

★ Has there been a change in setting?

★ Am I less active than normal?

★ Has my sleep changed?

★ Am I feeling more stressed than usual?

Take some time to figure out what has changed that has led to the gradual weight gain. Have you returned to previous lifestyle habits (the #1 reason most people regain weight)? If so, revisit the weight management tools that have worked for you in the past and implement them back into your routine.

However, at times, changing your behaviour for weight loss doesn't feel possible. You may not have the time or energy to dedicate to it, and it slips down the priority list. If this is the case, be kind to yourself and aim to choose nourishing foods that make you feel well and take a break from creating change. Set yourself a date to revisit making changes and perhaps share this with someone so you can be accountable. Goal setting is a great way to jump back in, or try some new recipes from one of the many Carbs & Cals BOOKS.

The strategy used for weight maintenance is often linked to the method you used to lose weight. The following section has guidance on how to adapt the different weight loss methods to go into the weight maintenance phase. However, it's worth reading them all, as you might pick up some new ideas on how to keep your weight stable.

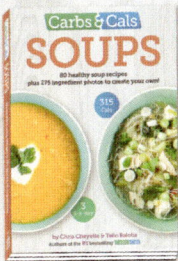

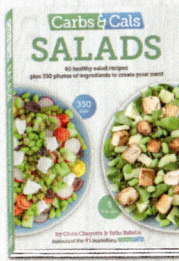

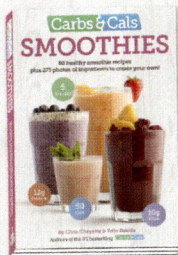

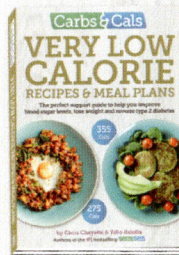

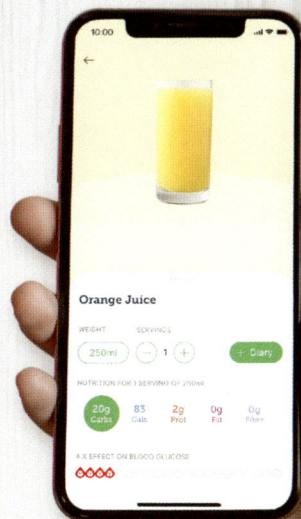

Calorie controlled diet

You may have reduced your daily calorie intake to 1800, 1500 or even 1200 calories in order to lose weight. Once you've achieved your target weight, you will be able to consume a higher amount of calories to keep your weight the same. There are a few options to do this:

Increase your daily intake by 300 to 500 calories, and keep monitoring your calorie consumption.

OR

Work out your personal calorie requirements to maintain weight using the BMI & Calorie Requirement Calculator (**www.carbsandcals.com/BMI**), and plan your daily intake to meet this target.

OR

Use your common sense and intuition to eat a bit more than you were in the weight loss stage. This could mean having a slightly larger portion, an additional snack in the day or allowing an extra treat or two each week.

In all cases, monitor your weight once a week at the same time of day, and adjust eating habits as necessary (i.e. cut back on calories a little if you notice weight going up consistently). Finding the balance between eating too much or not enough can take a little trial and error.

Very low calorie diet

Because the VLCD is usually followed for a set amount of time (3 months max), it has a clear start, middle and end. At this point, your healthcare professional will support you to transition from the weight loss period to a maintenance phase.

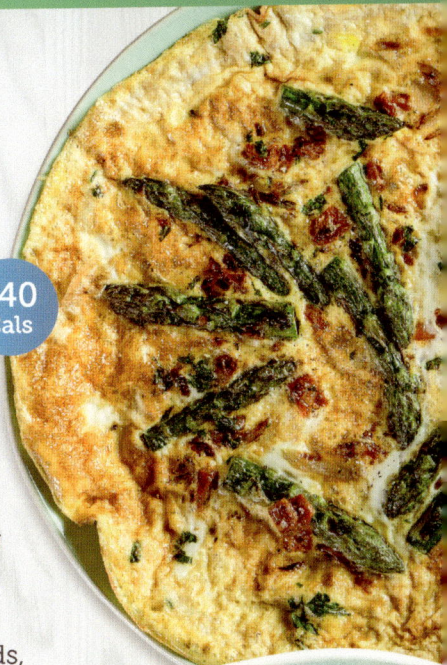

340 Cals

If you've been using shakes and supplements, this could mean introducing 1 meal a day alongside the shakes to gradually increase the daily calories. If you've been doing the VLCD with real foods, you can increase portion sizes.

The goal is to gradually increase the calories from the 800 target of the weight loss phase by 25% to 1000 calories, and then to 1200 and 1500 until reaching the amount you personally need to maintain weight (which you can work out at www.carbsandcals.com/BMI).

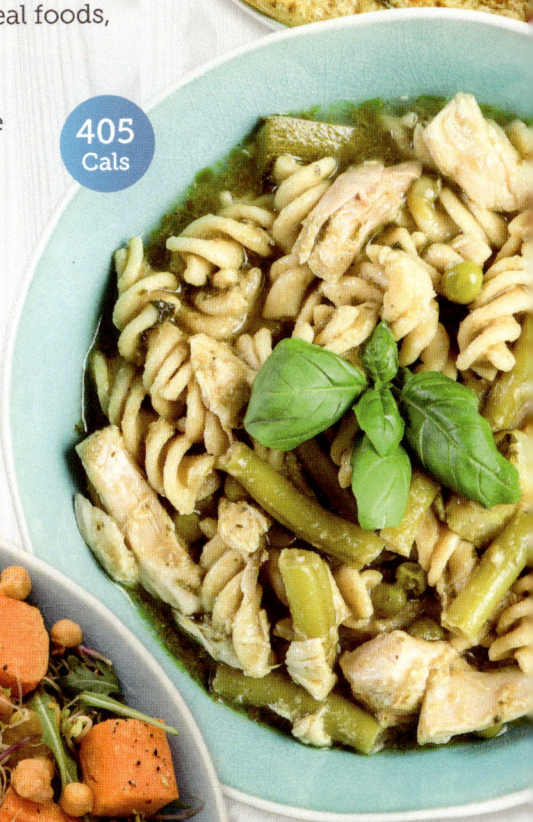

405 Cals

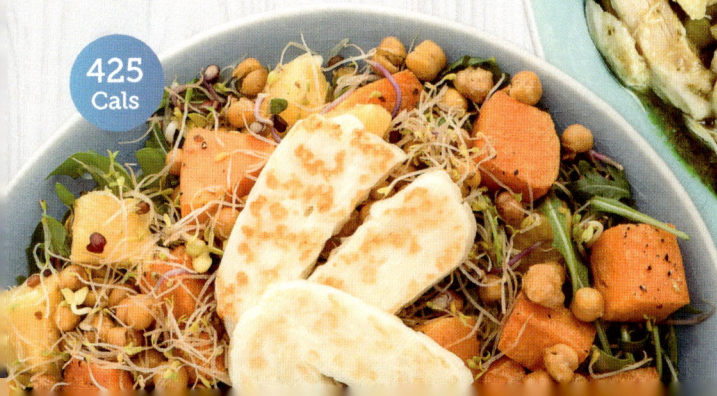

425 Cals

Intermittent fasting

Once you're in the swing of intermittent fasting, it can feel like the norm and carrying it on with a few small changes can be an easy way to maintain weight.

5:2

Switching from the 5:2 to a 6:1 fasting routine is a popular way of transitioning from weight loss to weight maintenance. Having just a single calorie-restricted fasting day per week increases your overall calorie intake compared to 2 fasting days, and gives you a little more flexibility.

16:8

You may find that the 16:8 works for your routine on an ongoing basis, and you're able to eat your meals within this timeframe without any feelings of deprivation. If this is continuing to keep your weight stable, keep calm and carry on!

However, if you're feeling restricted, give yourself a little more flexibility a couple of days a week (and on special occasions), to allow for a later dinner or earlier brunch. Alternatively, you could loosen the times to 14:10 to give you a 10 hour eating window with a little more breathing space.

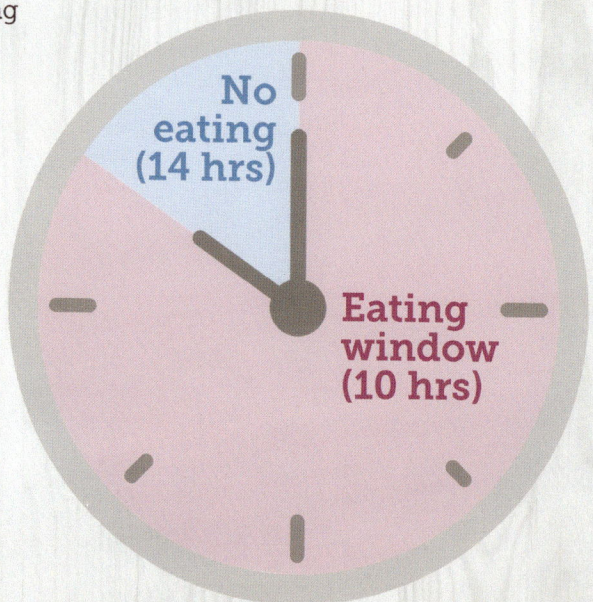

No eating (14 hrs)

Eating window (10 hrs)

Low carb diet

Research to support the use of a low carb diet for more than 12 months is minimal. This seems to be because most people find it difficult to follow this diet for long periods of time, but more research is needed. You may find it useful to use the low carb diet as a kickstart and then move to a moderate carb intake (130g to 230g carbs per day). No matter which approach you go for, focus on enjoying wholegrain and unprocessed carbs, and reducing white and refined carbs where possible.

Intuitive eating

If you've been successful with weight loss using the intuitive eating principles (see page 44 and 45) to achieve your target weight, you will have learned some valuable skills and changed your relationship with food. This new mindset puts you in a strong position for the weight maintenance phase. Continue to eat mindfully, monitor your weight regularly and adjust eating habits as necessary.

Physical activity

It is important to maintain physical activity no matter where you are in your weight loss journey. Regular exercise is also highly effective in long term weight management: many studies demonstrate that those that maintain or build their physical activity levels are more likely to maintain their lower weight. As well as helping you to lose weight, physical activity has many other benefits, including increased strength, lung capacity and mood!

Sticking to the new routine

Once you've reached your target weight and found an effective strategy to maintain it, the final challenge is to stick to the healthy eating habits and mindset that have got you this far. However, there are bound to be days where you veer off track, so having the awareness that this is happening and not letting it become a frequent occurrence is key.

For example, you've reached your target weight and you've built in 1 packet of crisps per week into your weight maintenance plan, but one evening you eat a large sharing bag all to yourself.

170 Cals

If we look at the bigger picture, that 1 large packet of crisps is over 750 calories. If this is not a regular occurrence, it's unlikely to have an impact on your long term goal. Don't be discouraged - simply refocus to keep yourself on track.

770 Cals

Some people find it helpful to keep a list of their food change achievements, by recording the changes they have made. Then, when they have a day that did not go to plan, they can refer back to the list to remind them of how far they have come. This can be a great tool to get back on track with your goals, and help boost confidence.

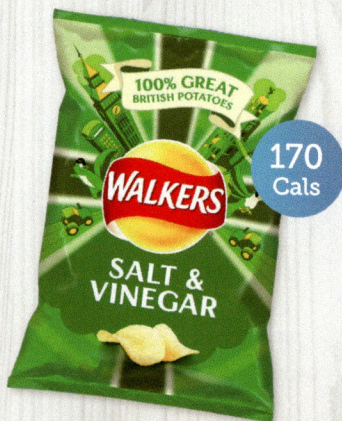

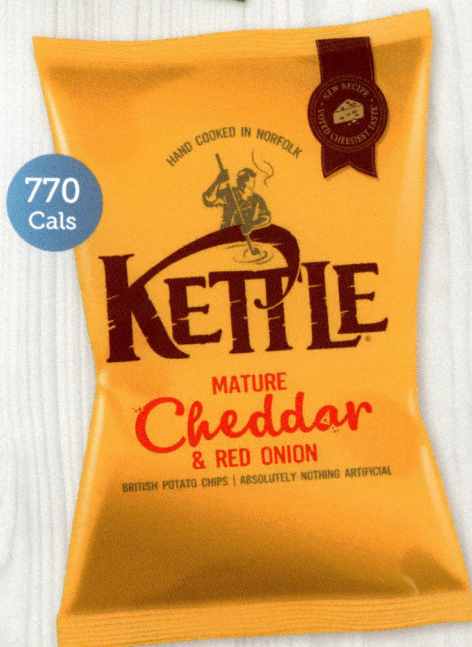

However, when these extras happen more often than you realise, your average daily calories may creep above the amount you need to maintain your weight, and this is what causes weight gain to start. To nip it in the bud, have a think about why the behaviour is happening. Ask yourself:

Are you eating enough during the day?

Is your weight maintenance strategy realistic and appropriate?

If you gave yourself permission to have 2 small packets of crisps per week, would that be enough to deter you from bingeing the large sharing bag?

Does it happen when you're feeling bored or tired?

Is it going hand-in-hand with a regular movie night or a catch up with friends?

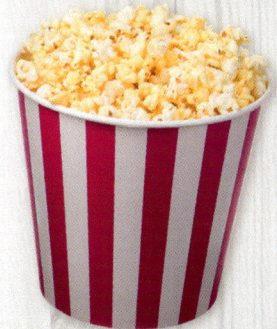

Remember, one indulgence doesn't mean failure or that you've let anybody down. If it's turning into a habit, explore it a bit more and see what you need to get back on track. Here are a few tips:

★ If it's hunger leading to that large snack, have a look at your routine on that day and enjoy more veggies, wholegrain carbs and protein with your meals so you feel more satiated later on in the day. Revisit your routine and check you are eating regularly enough to avoid unplanned snack attacks!

★ It's common to confuse hunger and thirst, so make sure you drink enough fluids throughout the day and evening. If you feel hungry, try having a glass of water or other low calorie drink first, to see if that solves it!

★ If the craving is driven by emotion, how can you deal with this without using food? For example, if it's boredom, think about what you enjoy doing: create some art, call a friend for a catch up, read a book or magazine, or go for a walk. You could even tick a few chores off the list to keep you busy!

★ If it's a social situation like a movie with friends, get into the habit of preparing healthier snacks like Kale Crisps or Spicy Chickpeas. These will still be crunchy and tasty, but much higher in fibre, and lower in salt and fat - giving you a similar snacking experience but in a healthier way.

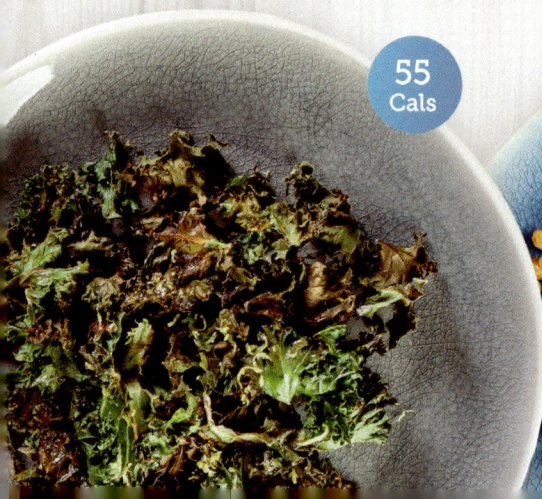

55
Cals

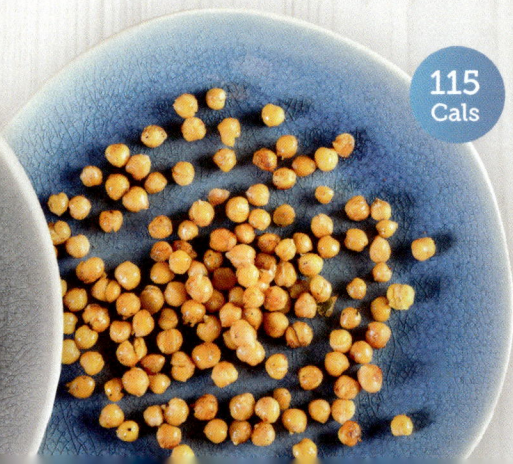

115
Cals

About the Authors

Will Hadfield MNutr RD & Emma Jones BSc (Hons) RD

Will and Emma are both Diabetes Specialist Dietitians, and have over 10 years experience each in the NHS, not-for-profit and freelance sectors working with people with diabetes. They formed their company, WE Nutrition (**www.wenutrition.co.uk**), to offer people an individual and tailor-made nutrition therapy service in the comfort of their own home. Their specialist skills and experience are used to help people achieve their health goals. They work with people, their families and with companies in all areas around nutrition, health and diabetes.

Chris Cheyette BSc (Hons) MSc RD
Diabetes Specialist Dietitian

Chris has over 20 years experience working with people with type 1, type 2 and gestational diabetes within the NHS. He is a co-creator of Carbs & Cals and is widely published in academic journals on diabetes and weight management. Chris lectures at national conferences and regularly appears in the media as a respected nutrition specialist.

Yello Balolia BA (Hons)
Creative Entrepreneur

Having achieved a first class honours degree in Photography, London-based Yello used his entrepreneurial and creative skills to found Chello Publishing Limited with Chris Cheyette, to publish Carbs & Cals (**www.carbsandcals.com**), the bestselling and award-winning book and app for diabetes and weight management.

Awards

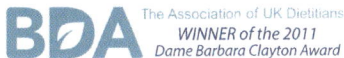
BDA The Association of UK Dietitians WINNER of the 2011 Dame Barbara Clayton Award

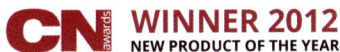
CN awards WINNER 2012 NEW PRODUCT OF THE YEAR

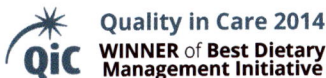
QiC Quality in Care 2014 WINNER of Best Dietary Management Initiative

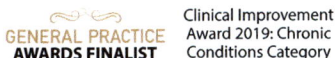
GENERAL PRACTICE AWARDS FINALIST Clinical Improvement Award 2019: Chronic Conditions Category

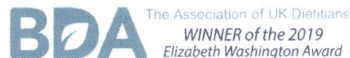
BDA The Association of UK Dietitians WINNER of the 2019 Elizabeth Washington Award

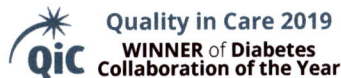
QiC Quality in Care 2019 WINNER of Diabetes Collaboration of the Year

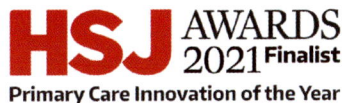
HSJ AWARDS 2021 Finalist Primary Care Innovation of the Year

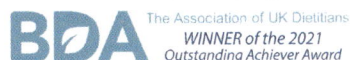
BDA The Association of UK Dietitians WINNER of the 2021 Outstanding Achiever Award

MORE FROM Carbs & Cals

Visual resources for diabetes, weight loss & healthy eating

WORLD FOODS

★ 750 photos of food & drinks from African, Arabic, Caribbean & South Asian communities

★ Uses new 'blood glucose icons' to show food's possible effect on blood glucose levels

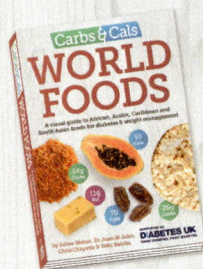

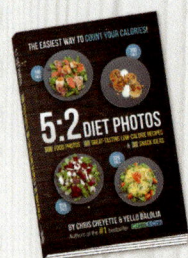

5:2 DIET PHOTOS

★ Delicious inspiration for 500 calorie fasting days

★ 600 photos, 60 recipes and 30 snack ideas

RECIPE BOOKS

★ 80 great tasting recipes per book

★ All recipes calorie & nutrient counted

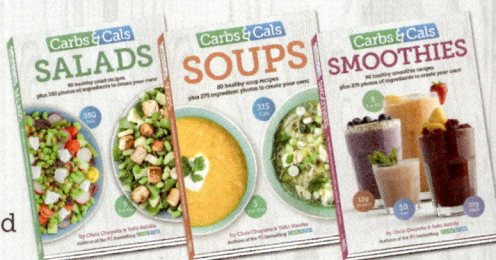

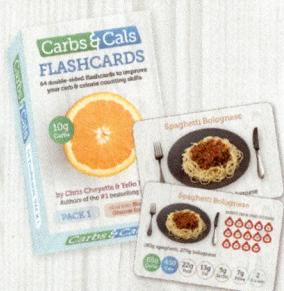

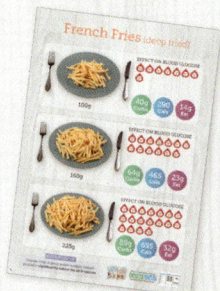

FLASHCARDS & POSTERS

★ 3 packs of 64 flashcards - ideal for teaching

★ Set of 10 handy A3 posters with common foods

50 FREE HEALTH RESOURCES

★ Register at www.carbsandcals.com/register

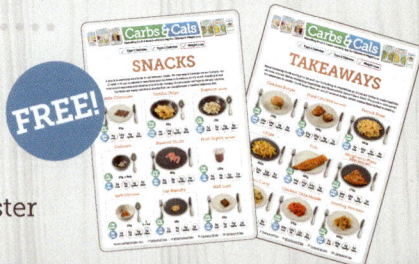

FREE!